HEA
THE ONLY
The Alternative

Written and Published by
Ian Sinclair
5 Ivy St
Ryde NSW
Australia 2112

First Edition 1995
Second Edition 2000
Third Edition 2002

ISBN 0-646-22643-6

Bt the same Author
Vaccination The 'Hidden' Facts
You Can Overcome Asthma

Order Details
www.vaccinationdebate.com
ian@vaccinationdebate.com

***"Make not authority your truth,
but instead,
make truth your authority".***

CONTENTS

Author's Introduction..1

1. Understanding Health..10

2. The Laws of Health..15

3. The Hopewood Children..20

4. Understanding Sickness..22

5. Vaccination - What it's really about...........................31

6. Questions and Answers..36

AUTHOR'S INTRODUCTION

On June 25th 1984, my son Robbie Jay was born. As neither my wife or myself knew much about parenthood and baby care, we relied very much on advice from baby Health Clinics and the local GP. Whilst we accepted most advice without question, I was hesitant on the issue of vaccination.

Several years earlier I had read Ross Horne's book 'The Health Revolution' in which he mentioned the polio vaccination disasters in the US and Canada. That stuck in my mind, so when the time came for Robbie Jay's first vaccinations I decided to hold off. In fact, I held off vaccinating Robbie Jay for a year, but finally, due to the continual prompting from the local health council, I took him for his first shots.

Three weeks after those first shots, he developed an acute skin condition known as eczema, which required hospitalisation. At the time, it never occurred to me that my son's illness may have been caused by the vaccinations. In hospital, he was treated with corticosteroid creams and bandaged from head to toe so that the only visible part of him were his eyes. Whilst he was in this condition, I was asked by one of the doctors caring for him, for permission to give him the whooping cough vaccine. The doctor told me that there was a whooping cough epidemic in the area, and that if he was not vaccinated, he could easily get the disease and die.

Again, there were doubts in my own mind, but without sufficient knowledge and understanding of vaccinations, I could only hope that allowing my son to be given the whooping cough injection was the right thing to do. So without much hesitation, I granted the doctor permission. My son, suffering from a very acute illness, and being treated with corticosteroid drug therapy, was injected with the whooping cough vaccine.

As fate would have it, the very day after this vaccination, I was browsing through a library in a Naturopathic college in Sydney, when I came across a British health magazine called 'Here's Health' (March 1980). The magazine contained an article titled 'Whooping Cough Immunisation: Why Professor Stewart opposes it'. Professor Stewart was a Scottish Professor of Medicine who had been involved in vaccination campaigns in the UK since 1947, and was considered a leading expert on the subject.

In his article, Professor Stewart first stated that he did not believe the vaccine was effective, and pointed out that in whooping cough outbreaks in both England and United States, around 50% of whooping cough cases occurred in fully vaccinated children. He further stated that the vaccine had never been proven to be adequate in protecting infants below one year of age, which he believed, were the only group of children whose health could be seriously menaced by whooping cough.

Professor Stewart claimed that the vaccine was dangerous and that hundreds if not thousands of well infants had suffered irreparable brain damage because of the vaccine. In his concluding comments, Professor Stewart stated, *"My own view, based upon some years of observation and experience, is quite firm. I supported the use of vaccine in 1951 and subsequently with very little hesitation until about 1972, and gave pertussis (whooping cough) vaccine between 1951 and 1956 to each of my four children. I would not dream so of doing again because it has become clear to me not only that the vaccine is incompletely protective, but also that the side-effects which I thought to be temporary are in fact dangerous, unpredictably so".*

Needless to say, after reading that article, my confidence and trust in the medical system was severely shaken. What bothered me the most was why the doctor who advised me to vaccinate Robbie Jay against whooping cough, made no mention of its risks or ineffectiveness. As I was to eventually learn, few doctors are truly aware of the risks or dangers associated with vaccines, let alone their ineffectiveness. Their knowledge is largely based on their university education and Drug Company literature, neither of which provide them with the true facts on vaccination. What's more, doctors do very little research into the scientific literature on vaccinations and are therefore unaware of the overwhelming evidence exposing their ineffectiveness and dangers. Worst of all, most doctors, conservative by nature and afraid of stepping out of line, will simply not open their eyes to the truth. It's far more comfortable and safer to follow the established order without question. Therefore, when it comes to the subject of Vaccination, I can say to you with absolute certainty, your doctor DOESN'T know best. (the few doctors who do research vaccination, often become its biggest critics, refer 'DOCTORS CONDEMN VACCINATION' in back pages).

As a result of reading Professor Stewart's article, I began researching vaccination, and for six years studied and researched medical journals, scientific literature and many books on vaccination. Briefly, this is what I discovered:-

- Graphical and statistical evidence showing that in excess of 90% of the decline in death rates from infectious disease occurred BEFORE vaccination commenced. All medical journals acknowledged this decline to improved sanitation, hygiene, better nutrition and living standards. In other words, vaccination was not responsible for wiping out infectious disease as medical authorities claim.

- That in the USA, despite compulsory vaccination, major outbreaks of measles and whooping cough were occurring amongst fully vaccinated children. In the UK since 1970, over 200,000 cases of whooping cough had occurred in fully vaccinated children.

- That a tuberculosis vaccine trial in India involving over 260,000 Indians (one of the largest vaccine trials ever conducted) resulted in more cases of TB amongst the vaccinated than the un-vaccinated. In simple terms, this meant that the tuberculosis (BCG) vaccine was totally useless. This vaccine is still being given to Australian children.

- That almost every polio case in the USA in the previous 30 years had been associated with the vaccine itself, the same vaccine given to all Australian children.

- That the cost of the whooping cough vaccine had risen from 11 cents in 1982 to $11.40 in 1987. The vaccine company was putting aside $8.00 per shot to cover legal costs and damages being paid out to parents of brain damaged children and children who died after vaccination.

- That between 1955 and 1984 over 200 million children were injected with contaminated polio vaccines containing the SV 40 virus, which were found to cause cancer in animals, as well as changes in human cell tissue cultures.

- That America's number one AIDS researcher, Dr. Robert Gallo, had speculated that the AIDS explosion was triggered by the World Health Organisation's smallpox campaign throughout Africa, Haiti and Brazil.

- That a survey in the UK involving over 600 doctors revealed that 50% of them refused the Hepatitis B vaccine despite belonging to the high risk group urged to be vaccinated. Amongst the reasons given for their refusal were *"I do not trust the vaccine"* and *"Vaccination is of no proven benefit"*.

- That millions of children in third world countries were still dying from measles, tuberculosis, diphtheria, tetanus, polio etc. DESPITE being fully vaccinated.

I must emphasise that most of the evidence I found exposing the ineffectiveness and dangers of vaccination were from medical sources, in most cases, medical journals or articles written by medical scientists and researchers. What this meant was that medical authorities knew this information but kept it from the public. It became clear to me that you could not rely upon medical authorities to provide accurate or truthful information about vaccination. I had gathered a large body of evidence which clearly proved that vaccines were not responsible for the eradication of infectious diseases as medical authorities claimed, that vaccines were neither safe nor effective, and that information handed out by Medical Authorities and Health Departments was fraudulent and misleading.

In order to get this evidence out to other parents and the public at large, I wrote and published the book 'Vaccination The Hidden Facts' in 1992. This book is currently sold and distributed throughout Australia, New Zealand, England and America. Copies can be obtained through mail order.

Between September 1993 and November 1994 I travelled throughout the Eastern States of Australia delivering lectures on the dangers and ineffectiveness of vaccines, along with a presentation of Natural Health philosophy on the prevention of childhood illness. All told, I covered approximately 95 towns and not one occasion was the evidence I presented ever challenged. In a number of towns, vaccine supporters attended my lectures, but did not refute the evidence or arguments presented. Throughout my journey I had an open challenge, still current today, for any doctor or health authority to debate vaccination publicly. At the time of this writing it has yet to be accepted.

Throughout Australia and many other countries there is a growing awareness of the dangers and ineffectiveness of vaccines. In Australia, this is evidenced by the formation of vaccine information groups that are providing the public with information on the risks associated with vaccines and evidence of their ineffectiveness. This is an extremely important and essential task and I applaud all of those organisations who are endeavouring to inform the public. However, informing the public of the dangers and ineffectiveness of vaccines is still only half the job. The most common question I was asked at my seminars and radio interviews was, *"well if vaccines don't work, what's the alternative?"*.

As parents become more aware of the pitfalls of vaccination, they will for obvious reasons seek an alternative approach to safeguard their children's health. A number of alternatives are now being offered parents, amongst them, homeopathic protection, vitamin therapy, improved nutrition and healthier lifestyle. Many parents are now choosing not to vaccinate their children, but are unsure as to the correct alternative. Some parents believe it is simply best to do nothing and if the child contracts an infectious disease, then it should be allowed to run its course. Parents who take this action generally see the infection as being beneficial in that it strengthens the body's natural immunity. Having spoken to many hundreds of parents throughout my seminars, I have found there to be a lot of uncertainty about the best alternative to vaccination.

It is this uncertainty and confusion over alternatives to vaccination that has prompted me to write this book. I believe that a genuine alternative does exist, an alternative that is both safe and effective, that will guarantee 100% protection from infectious disease, and that costs nothing. What is this alternative? HEALTH - THE ONLY IMMUNITY there is!

It is the purpose of this book to show you very clearly that there is only one type of immunity against disease, and one type only - HEALTH. In a state of true physiological health, I will show you that sickness cannot arise. I will show you that measles, whooping cough, polio and all the other infections cannot develop in a truly healthy body. In fact, I will go one step further and show you that NO DISEASE can develop in a HEALTHY body. But before I do this, I must take you back to 1984.

In February of that year, I enrolled at the NSW College of Natural Therapies to undertake Diploma courses in Nutrition and Therapeutic Massage. It was whilst researching in the college library that I came across a number of books and cassettes on Natural Health science. This science, also known as Natural Hygiene, was the basis of the biggest selling health book in history 'Fit For Life' which has sold over 9 million copies world wide.

Natural Health teaches you how to build and maintain high level health through the principles of natural living. Natural Health also teaches you how to prevent disease without vaccines and overcome disease without drugs. It's worth noting that the pioneers of Natural Health, were in actual fact medical doctors who discovered a non-drug approach in treating sickness. So successful were these doctors, that they abandoned their drug treatments altogether, and adopted the non-drug methods of Natural Health. One such doctor was R.T. Trall. In the USA in 1860, at a time when deaths from infectious disease exceeded 50% under medical treatment, Dr. Trall delivered a lecture at the famous Smithsonian Institute where he stated: *"I have myself, during the sixteen years that I have practised the Hygienic system, treated all forms and hundreds of cases of typhus and typhoid fevers, pneumonia's, measles and dysentery's, and have not lost a patient of either one of these diseases. And the same is true of scarlet and other fevers. And several of the graduates of my school have treated these cases for years, and none of them, so far as I know or have heard, have ever lost a patient when they were called in the first instance, and no medicine whatever had been given"*.

The basic principles of Natural Health have indeed been recognised and endorsed by some of the greatest minds in history. Amongst them, Pythagoras, Socrates, Plato, Hippocrates, Albert Einstein, Leonardo da Vinci, Benjamin Franklin, Thomas Edison, Voltaire, George Bernard Shaw and Mahatma Gandhi just to mention a few. In fact, if you were to study the lifestyles of those people throughout history who have demonstrated the highest levels of longevity, health and freedom from disease, you would find that their lifestyles were closely aligned to the teachings of Natural Health.

The great beauty of Natural Health is its simplicity and common sense, for unlike medical science with its complex theories and language, it is easily understood by the layman. The only difficulty that I experienced in the acceptance of these teachings was in changing my belief system. Up until I discovered Natural Health, my understanding of disease was based entirely upon the medical idea that germs or other outside influences were solely responsible, and that my only means of preventing or curing illness was through drugs or vaccines. Like most people, I was programmed with these beliefs since childhood, and as I soon learnt, long held beliefs are not always easy to remove.

I should also mention that being an asthmatic for most of my childhood and teenage years, and completely reliant on doctors and drug therapy, I was very conditioned to medical theories and ideas, so again, the acceptance of Natural Health theory, which is very much contrary to medical theory, was not immediately achieved. This probably explains why in 1985, having studied Natural Health for over a year, I still chose to have my son vaccinated.

Fortunately, life has a way of slapping you in the face in order to teach you something. The hospitalisation of my son following vaccination, and the return of my asthma that I thought I had outgrown many years earlier, were the two events in 1985 that proved to be the slap in the face I needed. I did not want a sick son, nor did I want to go through the suffering of asthma that I experienced as a child. So rather than just read or study Natural Health, I began to embrace and follow these teachings in my own life. I figured the best way to determine the truth of Natural Health theory was to put it to the test, after all, the greatest teacher in the world, is personal experience, is it not?

And thank God I did! For nearly ten years now I have followed the teachings of Natural Health. Now I don't mean that I've been an absolute puritan in all that time, there have been many occasions where I have fallen off the path for a while. Let's face it, we all like to party now and again. Yet in those ten years I have never been to a doctor, have taken no medical drugs whatsoever and have not spent one single cent on any sort of health care. On the few occasions that I've experienced sickness, which have usually coincided with those times when I've fallen off the path, I have taken no drugs and recovered quickly under Natural Health principles, which in most cases, involves nothing more than rest, fresh air and pure water.

Today, at 40 years of age, I no longer suffer from asthma or any of the other debilitating illnesses that plagued my childhood and teenage years.

In the case of Robbie Jay, since the day he left hospital almost ten years ago, he has never since been vaccinated, has never been to a doctor, nor has he even taken any drugs or antibiotics whatsoever. He has never even taken an aspirin or panadol. And again, I have not spent one single cent on my son's health care. Like myself, he has had a few bouts of sickness, mainly childhood fevers. In each case he has quickly recovered full health after a period of two to three days in bed with only pure water at his bedside. Today, at ten years of age,

Robbie Jay is a healthy, robust and fun-loving child.

Now the reasons I've talked about my experience over the past ten years is so you know what my qualifications are in writing this book. If I've learnt anything over that period of time, it is that you cannot learn or understand health merely through academic study or intellectual debate. Although I spent three years studying at a Naturopathic College, and did a couple of years correspondence study in physiology and nutrition, most of my understanding of Natural Health has come through living it and not just from textbook study. I firmly believe that if one is to know and understand health, then one must possess health.

My own experience and that of my son; ten years of research, study and investigation; scientific evidence and clinical results; common sense and logicality; it is all these things that has convinced me that the teachings of Natural Health are true and correct, and that only by adherence to these teachings can the health of our children be assured.

I have said that health is the only immunity there is. For this reason, I must commence by explaining to you what a HEALTHY body is. It will be necessary for me to take you inside the body so that you can understand what true physiological health is all about. This explanation will be presented in **Chapter 1**.

In **Chapter 2** you will learn about those simple laws which govern the health of the body. Obeyance to these laws will ensure radiant health in yourselves and your children.

In **Chapter 3** you will read about the Hopewood children, an inspiring example of the benefits of Natural Living.

In **Chapter 4** we will examine Natural Health theory on the causes of disease, how the symptoms of acute infectious disease are really beneficial, and the reasons why Natural Health rejects drugs and vaccines.

In **Chapter 5** we'll have a grandstand look at what vaccination is really about and the true motives behind it.

In **Chapter 6** I answer some of the most commonly asked questions on vaccination and Natural Health.

Like my previous books, this book is written specifically for the layman, and not for the academic or scientific minded. Readers with an academic interest, or who are seeking scientific reference should also research those books listed in bibliography.

In writing about Natural Health, I wish to emphasise that I am not seeking to preach, or to convert. Natural Health is not a religion, it is not a biblical doctrine, it is not a *'thou must live this way'* philosophy. Natural Health does not employ fear or guilt tactics to coerce you into accepting its teachings.

It is not my intention to lay it upon you in any way, for I believe that all people have the right to choose for themselves, their own type of lifestyle, the type of food they shall eat, whether they wish to smoke, drink or whatever. The right to think for ourselves and make our own choices in life is a God given right and a spiritual imperative. Let no one ever remove that right.

When I write about Natural Health, I'm not seeking to preach, but to inform, to increase awareness, to present truth, to bring light where there is darkness, and hopefully, to inspire where there is despair. I write about Natural Health not only because I believe it to be true, but because it exposes the erroneous theories of medical science, the criminal practice of vaccination and the insidious dangers of drug therapy.

Finally, in writing about Natural Health, I choose not to compromise these teachings, but to write of them in their true and ideal form. I do this for a very important reason. Many people who read this book, will do so because they are seeking direction. What better direction is there, than to know what the ideal is, and then strive to move towards it? The great beauty of an ideal, is that it gives you direction, and that is the primary purpose of this book.

Ian Sinclair
February 1995

1

UNDERSTANDING HEALTH

If you do not want your children to get measles, whooping cough, rubella, polio, or any of the other infections, then you must ensure that their bodies are HEALTHY. If you do not want your children to suffer from asthma, skin disease, allergy complaints or any other illness, then again, you must ensure that their bodies are HEALTHY. If YOU do not wish to suffer any illness, then keep your body HEALTHY. I have stated in the introduction that a healthy body cannot and does not get sick. Therefore, let us start by examining the physiological requirements for HEALTH.

1. The body must have all its necessary parts, and they must be in proper working order. In other words, the body must possess a brain, heart, lungs, kidneys, immune system, reproductive organs, etc. and they all must work. There must therefore be no genetic or hereditary defects.

2. There must be correct spinal alignment and muscular balance.

3. All the necessary nutrients such as glucose, fatty acids, amino acids, vitamins and minerals etc. must be present in adequate quantities to satisfy the body's needs for energy, growth, repair and maintenance.

4. The blood must be of the correct alkalinity which is approximately 7.4 pH.

5. The body's internal environment, both inside and outside the cells, must be free of accumulated toxins and waste material. In other words, the inside of the body must be CLEAN and HYGIENIC.

6. Above all else, the body must be charged with VITALITY. Vitality is to the body what electricity is to the computer. Vitality is what keeps the body alive and functioning, it is the power source of all cellular activity, in fact, vitality is LIFE. Vitality is a force or an energy that we take in through breathing and from absorption of the sun's rays. Often referred to as life-force, prana, chi, cosmic energy, etc., it is stored in the body's nervous system and certain glands, where it is then transmitted to all the cells of the body. From the book 'Hunza Health Secrets' author Renee Taylor writes, *"It is true that the*

PHYSIOLOGICAL HEALTH

All Parts Working

Spinal Health

Muscular Balance

Adequate Nutrients

Alkaline Bloodstream

Clean & Hygienic

HIGH VITALITY

"Perhaps the greatest want of our age, is a correct knowledge of the physiology of our being and the laws that govern life, health and disease".

Herbert Shelton

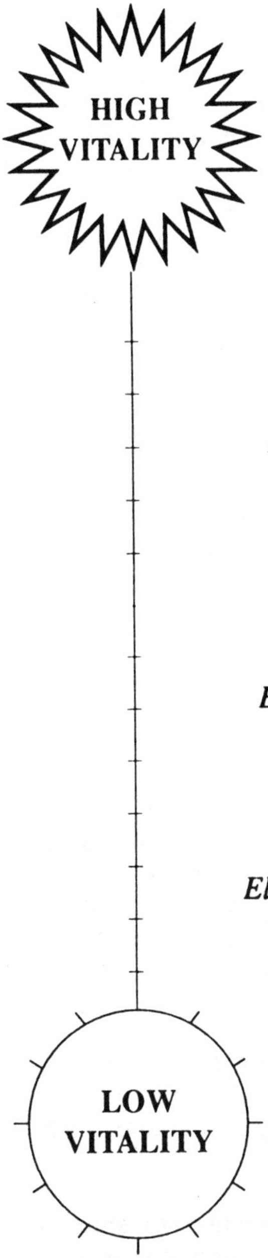

Imaginative

Creative

Inspired

Cheerful

Optimum Healing

Physically Strong

Perceptive

Mental Alertness

Powerful Intellect

Abundant Energy

Acute Senses

Radiant Appearance

↑ *VITALITY*

Fruits & Salads
Pure Water
Fresh Air
Sunshine
Deep Breathing
Relaxation
Proper Sleep
Exercise
Healthy Environment
Positive Thoughts
Purpose & Direction
Meditation & Prayer

↓ *VITALITY*

Animal & Refined Foods
Impure Water
Stale Air
Lack of Sunshine
Shallow Breathing
Tension
Insufficient Sleep
Sedentary Living
Environmental Pollutants
Negative Thoughts
Boredom & Worry
Drugs & Vaccines
Cigarettes & Alcohol
Stimulants - Coffee etc.
Electromagnetic Radiation
Sexual Excesses

Dullness

Depression

Heaviness

Unhealthy Appearance

Slow Healing

Lethargy

Fatigue

Pain & Sickness

Low Energy

Sluggish Metabolism

body requires food, but it is a false assumption when we think we receive strength only from the food we eat. The body, collectively, consists of myriads of cells, each a body in itself, complete with head and brain. This little brain of the cells is technically known as the nucleus and consists primarily of gray matter.... This gray matter has the ability to store magnetic energy within itself. Thus in each and every one of our cells we can receive and store up potential cosmic energy". A high amount of this energy or vitality means the body will be stronger, healthier, mentally alert, imaginative, creative etc., whereas a low level of vitality means the body will be weak, more prone to sickness, mentally dull and lacking in imagination and creativity. VITALITY is the key to not just freedom from disease, but to optimum PHYSICAL and MENTAL HEALTH.

"..... the pleasure afforded by every organic form is in proportion to its appearance of healthy vital energy".

John Ruskin

As I have said before, and must now say again, in this state of health, in this state of TRUE PHYSIOLOGICAL HEALTH, sickness, measles, whooping cough, asthma, skin disease, infection, allergy, arthritis, candida, chronic fatigue, cancer, disease of whatever name is given to it, CANNOT and WILL NOT arise. No matter how many germs and viruses the body is exposed to, it is a physiological impossibility for sickness of any kind to arise when the body is in the state of health that has been described.

The common belief, fostered by medical theorists, is that the immune system is designed to fight off and destroy disease causing germs (viruses and bacteria). The idea of vaccination is to make the immune system stronger so that it be more effective in fighting off germs. The fallacy of this theory is exposed when one learns the true biological role of germs in the body, that it is not open warfare between germs and the immune system, but one of peaceful coexistence. Germs consume organic wastes undergoing decay, thereby aiding in the important task of keeping the system clean. As you will learn in **Chapter 4 - Understanding Sickness,** it is the build-up of toxic wastes or a polluted body that creates infection and disease within the body.

Real immunity against disease is a state of physiological health. The primary purpose of your immune system is to keep your system clean, to neutralise and destroy foreign material that is floating throughout the body. If you have a clean and hygienic system, if your bloodstream is pure, if there is no accumulated rubbish within your tissues, then you have immunity. This is the only type of immunity from disease there is, and is the only type of immunity you need.

In his book 'The Hygienic Care of Children', Herbert Shelton lists the leading characteristics of a normal, healthy, well-nourished child. They include *"Cheerfulness, bright sparkling wide open eyes, a good appetite, absence of vomiting, normal bowel movements, very little crying, perfect sound continuous sleep with eyes and mouth closed, symmetrical development of muscular and not fatty tissue, no evidence of pain or discomfort, and a clear skin with a peaches and cream complexion"*.

Regardless of age, those who possess true physiological health will not only be free from sickness and immune to all disease, but will demonstrate high levels of intelligence, imagination, creativity, perception and intuition. The signs of health include mental alertness, brightness, cheerfulness and a happy disposition. The healthy body will be strong, upright and firm in appearance, and there will be lightness and spring in every step. From his book 'Health Secrets Of All Ages' Eric Powell presents an inspiring description of health, *"When thinking is easy, when you can concentrate without difficulty and solve your problems as they turn up, when you are not conscious that you have a body, when you are free from aches and all physical distress, when you can stand, walk and run without being aware of your own weight, when you see beauty all about you, when living is a sheer joy, then you are in a state of health"*.

As important as it is for you to know what physiological health is all about, it is even more important to know the determinants of physiological health, or in other words, to know what are those things that are responsible for producing and maintaining a healthy body. So how do you ensure that your baby is born with a healthy body, how do you ensure health in your children, how do you ensure health in yourself?

The answer, I believe, is to know and understand those laws that govern the health of the body, and then as best you can, strive to live in accordance with them.

"Every man, women and child holds the possibility of physical perfection, it rests with each of us to attain it by personal understanding and effort"

F.M. Alexander

2

THE LAWS OF HEALTH

There is an old Chinese proverb that reads *"Those who disregard the Laws of Heaven and Earth have a lifetime of calamities, while those who follow the laws remain free from dangerous illnesses"*. Many volumes have been written on those natural laws which govern the health of all life, however, for the purposes of this book, they can be summarised and simplified so that they are easily understood.

Healthy Parents

It all starts with two healthy parents; two parents with HEALTHY bodies. Think about it. The father provides the seed, the mother the soil. Only healthy parents can produce a truly healthy baby.

Natural Childbirth

What better start to the health of the new born baby than to be born to a healthy mother, in the comfort and security of her own home, and to be placed in her arms immediately after birth. Just realise however, that the most important requirement for natural pain free childbirth is a HEALTHY mother. Many mothers because of their own poor health and large sized babies, are incapable of natural child birth and therefore require medical intervention (drugs, induction, forceps or caesarean delivery) which whilst necessary, are nevertheless injurious to both mother and child.

Breast Feeding

Everyone agrees that there is no better nourishment for the baby than breast milk from a healthy mother. Just realise however that the baby's digestive system is not ideally suited to solid foods until about two years of age. It is for this reason that Natural Health recommends breast feeding the baby for at least the first two years of life. When this is not possible, nut milk, juices, or goat milk should be substituted.

Live Food

The most ideal food for the human body, child or adult, is food from the PLANT KINGDOM. The human body is not carnivorous but frugivorous and is best nourished on a diet of fresh fruits, salad vegetables, grains and nuts. Such foods will provide all the protein, carbohydrates, fats, vitamins, minerals and trace elements needed for growth and energy, as well as maintaining an alkaline blood stream.

Pure Water

Clean, pure, unfluoridated, unchemicalised water, H20. Seventy percent of your body is water, if you want a clean pure body, make sure your drinking water is clean and pure.

Fresh Air and Sunshine

That VITALITY I mentioned in the last chapter, that energy or life-force that keeps the body healthy and strong, well it is to be found in the fresh air and sunshine. Do not take these for granted, fresh air day and night, and regular exposure to the sun's rays are essential for optimum health. Do not be afraid of the sun, its rays are health giving, just let common sense determine length of exposure.

Deep Breathing

One of the most powerful means of building up the vitality of the body. Through deep breathing you take into the system large quantities of this vitality, life-force, prana, also referred to a negative ions. This energy is then stored in your nervous system, glands and cells, providing your body with maximum electrical power.

Correct Posture

Stand tall, walk tall and sit tall. This practice helps to maintain correct spinal alignment and muscular balance, and is essential to proper breathing and the healthy functioning of the nervous system.

Exercise and Movement

Movement is as essential to the body, as swimming is to a fish. It is through movement that the muscles and bones are kept strong, that blood circulation and toxic elimination are stimulated, and that massage is given to the internal organs. Walking, dancing, swimming, aerobics, yoga, tai chi, etc. are all beneficial to the body and deserve their place in a regular daily routine.

Rest and Sleep

When it comes to restoring the vitality and recharging your battery, nothing is of more importance than rest and proper sleep. Sleep is the great rejuvenator, with no equal. Importantly too, it is during sleep that the body energies are most directed towards inner cleansing and repair, thus preserving bodily health.

Healthy Environment

An environment that is not only clean, hygienic and ecologically sound, but an environment that you are personally in harmony with. In other words, if you love the surf, don't live in the desert.

These then, are the physical laws that govern the health of the human body. I don't claim that they represent the complete list, nor do I claim that their explanations are complete. My main purpose was just to give you an awareness of what those major laws are and sufficient explanation for basic understanding. In those areas where you would like more information, e.g. natural childbirth, live food, etc. check out the recommended reading in the back of this book or consult your bookstore.

As I have learnt, it is no easy task being a parent. Yet, if you choose to have children, then you must accept the responsibility that goes with it. You cannot pass off this responsibility to your Doctor or your Naturopath. They can do nothing to build and maintain health in your children. That task can only be accomplished by the parents, so it is essential to understand these laws of health, and then do your very best to fulfil them. If there is one area in particular that I would emphasise, it is CORRECT DIET.

The ***ideal*** diet of both child and adult should consist of at least 80% fresh fruits and salad vegetables, with the remaining 20% consisting of whole grains, nuts and seeds. This diet will provide all the necessary protein, calcium, iron and other nutrients required for growth and energy. There are many books that provide enticing recipes based upon natural food selections that will appeal to children. With regard to animal and dairy foods, they are ruinous to health, in that they are to high in protein, fat, cholesterol, and contain large amounts of metabolic wastes, chemicals and drug residues. It is beyond the scope of this book to explain in detail the harmful effects of animal and dairy foods, however the best selling 'Fit For Life' or my book, 'You Can Overcome Asthma', offers a thorough explanation.

Having dealt very briefly with the PHYSICAL laws of health, I will be even more brief in dealing with those MENTAL and SPIRITUAL laws of health. The fact that I will only speak briefly of them should in no way imply that they are of any less importance. On the contrary, of all those laws which govern our health, none are of greater importance or have as much impact upon our health than those laws pertaining to MIND and SPIRIT.

The laws of mind and spirit are all to do with feelings, thoughts, attitudes, likes and dislikes, emotions and desires. They are about doing your thing, enjoying life and having fun. The laws of mind and spirit are about purpose, direction, focusing on one's goals and aspirations, developing and using your creative talents for service to humanity, and in so doing finding inner fulfilment and satisfaction. The laws of mind and spirit involve such things as non-judgement, non-criticism, respect, and compassion, allowing people to live their lives without infringing upon them, being honest and truthful, and simply learning to get along with all people regardless of colour, race or creed. The laws of mind and spirit are all about these things, and according to the ancient wisdom's, our sole purpose for being here is to learn them.

So how do these laws of mind and spirit impact our health? Let's keep it very simple. Remember that thing called VITALITY, the electrical energy of the body, the life-force which sustains all cellular activity. Remember that I said HIGH VITALITY keeps the mind and body strong, whereas LOW VITALITY leaves the body weak. Well, thoughts and feelings of a positive nature such as love, kindness, praise, compassion, contentment, joy, etc. have a strengthening and stimulating effect on the vitality of the body thus enhancing and maintaining health. On the other hand, thoughts and feelings of an opposite nature, e.g. anger, hatred, criticism, envy etc., have the reverse effect, weakening and draining the vitality of the body.

By understanding these laws of mind and spirit, you can appreciate that nourishment of the mind with good thoughts is just as important as nourishment of the body with good food. Many parents, myself included here, often concentrate so much on the physical requirements of diet, exercise, sleep, etc., for their children, that the spiritual needs of love, tolerance and patience etc., find only a back seat. Yet, of all those things which children most need to preserve their health, I would have to place at the top of the list, LOVE FOR YOUR CHILDREN.

An awareness of those physical, mental and spiritual laws that govern the physiological health of the body should enlighten you as to why there is so much sickness in our society. If you were to examine the lifestyle, eating habits, mental state etc., of any person (child or adult) afflicted with infectious disease, asthma, arthritis, chronic fatigue, cancer or any other disease, I do not believe you would find one single case, NOT ONE SINGLE CASE in which their lifestyle etc., was in harmony with the laws of health. Sickness is not bad luck, it is not the weather, it is not God's will and rarely is it karma. Sickness is a direct consequence of breaking those laws that govern the health of the body. The words of 17th century poet John Dryden are still true today. *"Look around the habitable world, how few know their own good, or knowing it, pursue"*.

I know that what I have written in this chapter is very ideal, but remember, the ideal gives you direction. Also, you should realise that the body is extremely strong and durable. The occasional junk-out, a few beers down the pub now and again, a couple of days being stressed out, etc., are not going to destroy your health, if for most of the time you are holding it together. It is not what you do 10% of the time, but what you do 90% of the time that determines your level of health. Nature is very forgiving, she gives us all a certain amount of leeway, but if we continually overstep her boundaries, then sickness and decay will be the consequence.

It is said that knowledge is power. By knowing what true health is all about, and by knowing and understanding those laws that govern health, you will realise that the power to build health, to maintain health, to protect health, or to restore health should it be lost, resides firmly within your own hands. Optimum health, high vitality, immunity from disease, these are the rewards to those whose lives are in harmony with Natural Laws. If health be your desire, if you are desirous of healthy children, then do the very best you can to follow these laws. The degree to which you are able to embrace them, will directly determine the degree of health that you and your children will enjoy. It is entirely in your hands, you have been given the tools, it's up to you whether you wish to use them.

***"Make mother nature your personal friend.
Here is a friend that will never, ever fail you
if you will work with her and not against her".***

3

THE 'HOPEWOOD' CHILDREN

In 1942 Mr. Leslie Owen Bailey, a great philanthropist and founder of the Natural Health Society of Australia, accepted guardianship of 85 children whose mothers were unable to care for them. Raised in accordance with Natural Health principles, and cared for in Hopewood House at Bowral, NSW, they were to become well known as the 'Hopewood' children.

Many of these children were young babies, and because breast feeding was not possible, they were reared on goats milk. The older children were initially given unpasteurised cows milk, but due to mucous problems in some children, fresh fruit and vegetable juices were substituted. From age two onwards, the diet of these children consisted of fresh fruit, root and green vegetables, salads, eggs, nuts, rice, porridge, wholemeal bread and biscuits, dried fruits, unsalted butter, lentils and soya beans etc. Between meals, only fruit or fruit juices were allowed, and children were encouraged to drink plenty of water, which, coming from the local water supply was pure and fluoride free. Treats consisted of 'Hopewood lollies' made from carob, coconut, dried fruits and honey.

The Child Welfare Department, who were overseeing the children's health insisted that the children be given 'meat', but when it was served to the children, they refused to eat it. Nutritionists from the Sydney University analysed the nutritional content of the Hopewood diet and the results showed adequate, even superior levels of protein, carbohydrate, fat and minerals in the food compared with orthodox diets. After the results of these tests were made known, the Child Welfare Department no longer insisted that the children be fed meat.

It is noteworthy that amongst these 85 children, no serious illness ever occurred, no operative treatments were ever performed, no drugs of any kind were ever taken or used, and NO VACCINATIONS were ever given. The only malady that occurred was when 34 of the children developed chicken pox. They were immediately put to bed and given only pure water or fresh fruit juice. They all recovered quickly without after-effects. Investigations revealed that these children whilst at school, had been swapping their healthy lunches for unhealthy conventional foods, so this outbreak was not altogether surprising.

In 1947, Dr. N.E. Goldsworthy, a medical doctor and head of the Institute of Dental Research in Sydney, wanted to investigate the dental health of the Hopewood children. Dr. Goldsworthy and his team conducted an extensive survey of the children's teeth over a 10 year period. This survey showed that the Hopewood children had 16 times less decay than other Sydney children the same age. Where Sydney children had on average 9.5 decayed, missing or filled teeth per child, there was only 0.58 in the Hopewood children. To use Dr. Goldsworthy's own words, the results were *"little short of miraculous"* The Hopewood children were credited with having the highest standard of dental health ever studied, even surpassing New Guinea native children who were supposed to have the best teeth in the world.

The Medical Profession also took an interest in the Hopewood children with Sir Lorimer Dodds and Dr. D. Clements, Head of Child Nutrition at Sydney University, monitoring their health for over 9 years. They examined both tonsils and adenoids and said they had never seen a group so free of trouble as the Hopewood children.

Many professional people visited Hopewood including Lord Mellamby of London (once physician to the Royal Family) and heads of dental research from the United Kingdom, USA, and New Zealand. Dr. Cumming from England was so impressed with the children's health that she gave many public lectures on their achievements. Child psychologist, Zoe Benjamin, an expert of the day, spent time with the Hopewood children and expressed amazement at their independent personalities and contentment as a group.

Most remarkable of all was the fact that many of these children inherited poor health due to a history of illness and malnourishment in their mothers. Despite this, and the fact that they were neither breast fed nor could enjoy the normal bonding of mother to child, they were able to grow into sturdy, self-reliant children.

The Hopewood children serve as an inspiring example for all of those parents who would like to raise their children 'naturally', and without, drugs and vaccines. These children are testimony to the truth and validity of Natural Health.

The full story of the Hopewood children appears in the Natural Health magazines Volume 5, No's 3;4;5;6 and Volume 6, No 1, published by the Natural Health Society of Australia (address in Bibliography).

4

UNDERSTANDING SICKNESS

If a child develops measles, mumps, whooping cough, rubella, or any of the other common childhood infections, then it is because that child does not possess a clean and healthy system. If a child develops skin disease, bronchial troubles, asthma, allergy disorders or any of the other common infantile diseases, then again it is because that child does not possess a clean and healthy system. If a child develops any of these sicknesses, then it is because that child's system is TOXIC or POLLUTED, a condition that Natural Health refers to as Toxaemia. (see diagrams on following pages).

Dr. Henry Bieler, author of 'Food is Your Best Medicine' writes *"The primary cause of disease is not germs. Disease is caused by a Toxaemia which results in cellular impairment and breakdown, thus paving the way for the multiplication and onslaught of germs".* Natural Health teaches that the root cause of most disease, including infection, is a toxic system, which they refer to as Toxaemia. Natural Health does not deny the presence of germs in infectious disease, but explains that their presence is a direct consequence of the toxic conditions of the body.

Toxaemia simply means that there is too much toxic waste material in the body. This waste material is made up of the body's own metabolic wastes together with foreign waste material such as chemicals, preservatives, insecticides, drug and vaccine residues, environmental pollutants etc. Whenever Toxaemia is present, there will often be accompanying disorders such as spinal lesions and subluxations, (unhealthy spine), nutritional deficiencies and sluggish metabolism. In most cases, simply having one of these conditions can lead to the others. In other words, a toxic system can cause spinal lesions; spinal lesions can cause nerve impingement; nerve impingement can result in sluggish metabolism; sluggish metabolism adversely affects digestion and assimilation of nutrients, leading to nutritional deficiency. (Each of these conditions can lead to the others). Just realise that if one part of the body is not healthy, or not working properly, then eventually, it will adversely effect the whole body.

"The smallest instrument out of tune
brings discord into the harmony of life".

Dr. Thomas Nichols

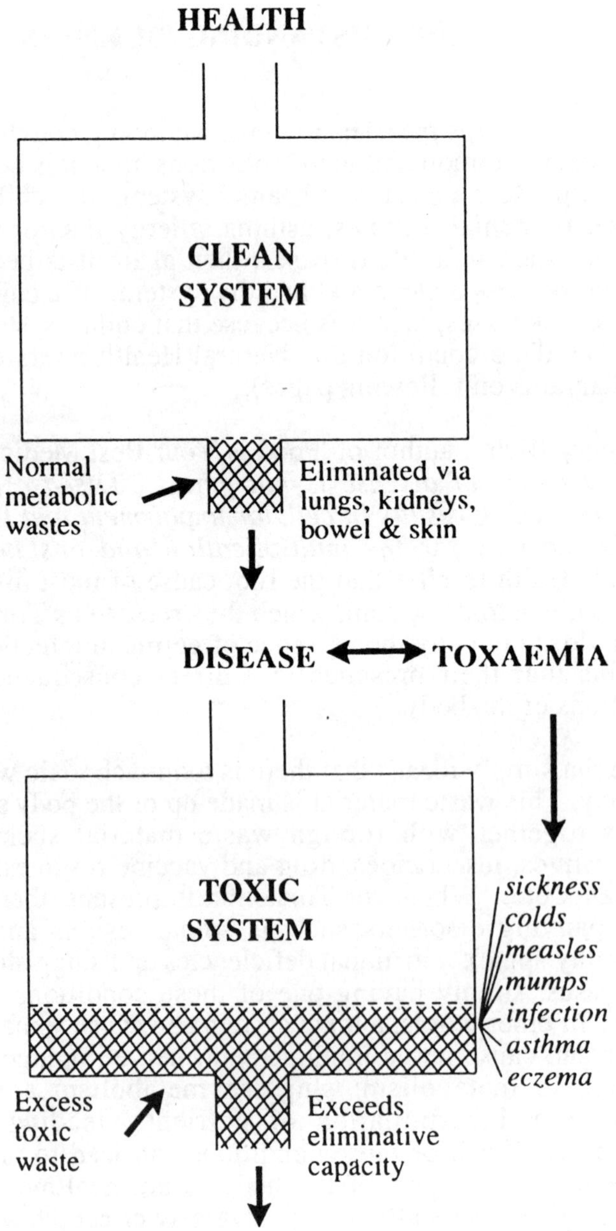
HEALTH
CLEAN SYSTEM
Normal metabolic wastes
Eliminated via lungs, kidneys, bowel & skin
DISEASE
TOXAEMIA
TOXIC SYSTEM
sickness
colds
measles
mumps
infection
asthma
eczema
Excess toxic waste
Exceeds eliminative capacity

Toxaemia and the Evolution of Disease

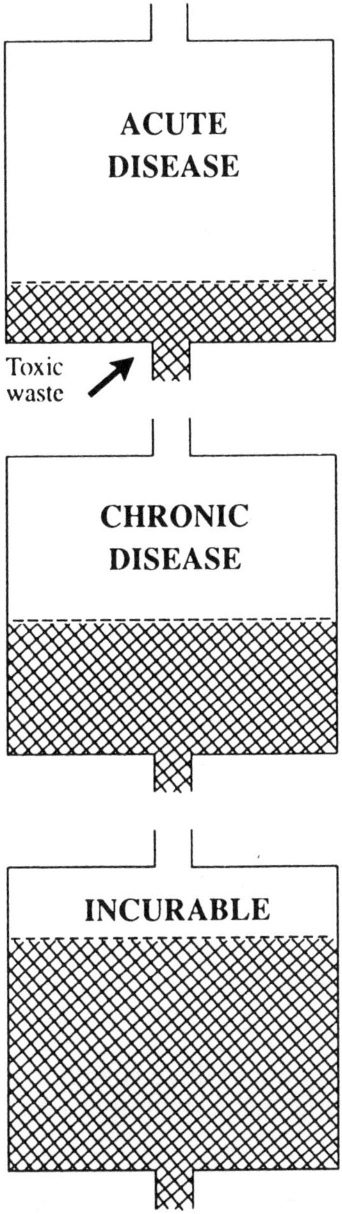

- fever, chicken pox, flu, tonsillitis, whooping cough, skin rashes, runny nose etc.

"...to check and suppress acute diseases means to suppress Nature's purifying and healing efforts, and to change the acute constructive reactions into chronic disease conditions."

Dr Henry Lindlahr

- arthritis, diabetes, ulceration, chronic fatigue, kidney disease, rheumatism etc.

"...the greatest part of all chronic disease is created through the suppression of acute disease by means of drug poisons and through the destructive effects of the drugs themselves."

Sir William Osler

- cancer and other malignant tumors (advanced stage)

"Cancer, tuberculosis, Bright's disease and all chronic diseases were once innocent colds...."

Dr J H Tilden

It is important that you understand the causes of Toxaemia, and the relationship between Toxaemia and disease. Let's start with the **Causes of Toxaemia.**

Low Vitality - all the mental, physical and physiological functions weaken and slow down. The immune system and eliminative organs which have the job of neutralising and eliminating toxic and metabolic wastes from the body, become sluggish and less efficient. The net result is a build-up of toxic waste within the blood and tissues. The causes of low vitality are numerous and include lack of fresh air and sunshine, shallow breathing, insufficient sleep, overwork, sedentary living, electromagnetic radiation, emotional stress, boredom, worry, overeating, medical drugs, etc.

Environmental and Chemical Pollutants - If the amount of chemicals and other pollutants that enter your body, exceed the amount that your body can eliminate, then again, the net result will be a build-up of toxic waste. The major causes are the conventional chemicalised diet, particularly animal, dairy and refined foods, fluoridated water (fluoride is a rat poison), drugs and vaccines, smoking, alcohol, and atmospheric pollutants.

Spinal Subluxations - the efficiency of all the metabolic processes including 'elimination' is dependent upon adequate nerve supply. Spinal subluxations, misalignment and lesions, or in simple terms, an unhealthy spine, will interfere and diminish proper nerve supply to the organs of the body. If the eliminative organs are affected, their performance will be impaired thus leading to a build-up of toxic waste. Subluxations can be caused by traumatic childbirth, weak muscular condition, poor posture, incorrect use of the body, accident or injury, lowered vitality, muscular imbalance and tension, etc.

Nutritional Deficiency - if the body is not supplied with all the necessary nutrients, if it is not getting enough vitamins and minerals, then every cellular activity, every metabolic function, in fact the whole system will begin to break down. This leads directly to Toxaemia. Causes of nutritional deficiency are numerous and include deficient diets, high protein diets, malnourishment, poor digestion and assimilation, lack of sunshine and medical drugs.

Putrefaction and Fermentation - any foodstuff within the digestive tract that has not been properly broken down and digested will soon begin to ferment and putrify. Not only can this result in bacterial or parasitic infection, but the end products of fermentation and putrefaction e.g. indol, skatol, methane gas etc., are poisonous and can be absorbed into the bloodstream thereby adding to the toxic waste level in the body. The main causes of fermentation and putrefaction can be traced to poor food combining, overeating (particularly flesh foods), drinking with meals, eating during acute illness and eating when under emotional stress.

You can see that the causes of Toxaemia are very much related to the orthodox lifestyle. Parents should realise that in babies and infants, toxaemia can easily develop through such things as polluted breast milk, fluoridated water, drugs and vaccines, powdered milk, over excitement, overeating, and lack of fresh air and sunshine. In fact, many babies are born with toxic systems because of poor parental health. Over 80 years ago, renowned British physician, Sir Arbuthnot Lane stated;

"There is but one cause of disease, poison toxaemia, most of which is created in the body by faulty living habits and faulty elimination".

Whilst it is easy to see the connection between unhealthy lifestyle and Toxaemia, it's not so easy to see how Toxaemia causes children's sickness such as the infectious diseases, or asthma, or skin disease, or any of the other diseases so common to children. How does Toxaemia actually cause these diseases?

Toxic waste matter is poisonous, its retention within the system will damage and ultimately destroy body tissues and cells unless removed. Fortunately, our bodies are equipped with a safety valve that enables the body to throw out excess toxic waste so as to ensure that it doesn't reach dangerous levels. What is this safety valve ? SICKNESS!

Whenever a child has a fever, sore throat, runny nose, no appetite, skin rash, mucous elimination, etc. then all it means is that the child is experiencing a cleansing reaction, an elimination of toxic waste that built up within its system. From the Natural Health viewpoint, acute sickness in children, such as measles, mumps, chicken pox, rubella or flu, is in reality, the body's efforts at eliminating excess toxic waste, and for this reason, is BENEFICIAL. This explains why children who develop acute sickness and are treated in accordance with Natural Health principles i.e. bed rest, pure water and fresh air, not only recover without suffering or complications, but are in better health afterwards. By allowing the sickness to run its course, their systems are cleansed, thus restoring their health.

Acute sickness, is not a mistake, it is not something evil, it is not the body being attacked by something outside itself, it is quite simply, a process of internal housecleaning. Over 2000 years ago, a man by the name of Hippocrates, who today is referred to as the Father of Medicine wrote *"Diseases are crises of purification, of toxic elimination"*.

On the other hand, when you treat children suffering these sicknesses with medical drugs, what you are basically doing, is closing that safety valve. You are preventing their bodies from eliminating all that toxic waste. This is what drug therapy does, it SUPPRESSES the body's attempts at cleansing its own system. In the western industrialised countries, one of the major reasons why some children suffer and die from these illnesses is because of suppressive drug therapy. If you know any child who has ever developed complications or died from any of these infectious diseases, just find out how the child was treated. When you hear of all those poor children in hospital suffering from whooping cough, realise that all of that suffering is directly due to the effects of suppressive drugs and wrong treatment. British Naturopath and Author, Harry Clements writes: *"It should always be borne in mind when thinking of complications, that they too often wait, not upon the original disease, but upon the treatment of it"*.

Now it's a different matter in third world countries where millions each year die of measles, diphtheria, whooping cough, etc., however, realise that their deaths are not due to these diseases, but to their own poor health brought about through malnourishment, starvation, impure water and unsanitary living conditions.

It is absolutely crucial that you understand this philosophy of disease as taught by Natural Health. If a child has measles, whooping cough, chicken pox, or any so called infectious disease, realise that the symptoms of these diseases i.e. fever, no appetite, lethargy, glandular swellings, skin rashes etc., all arise from the one underlying cause, Toxaemia, and all serve the same purpose, the elimination of toxic waste. Hippocrates taught *"All disease is one"*. All of the common infantile diseases, regardless of their name or type of symptoms, have as their root cause, Toxaemia. Hippocrates also wrote *"The symptoms of disease are evidence of the body's natural curative reactions"*. He is saying that the sickness is curative, or in other words, is BENEFICIAL. This is exactly what Natural Health teaches.

If this philosophy is new to you, if you've never read about Natural Health before, then you're probably still wondering where GERMS fit in to all of this. According to medical theory, which most people believe in, germs are the cause of sickness. Germs are what cause measles, polio, tuberculosis and infectious disease. Ever heard of Louis Pasteur? He was the scientist who came up with the Germ Theory of Disease over 100 years ago. Pasteur is to Medicine, what Christ is to the Church - their Saviour. Did you know that before Pasteur died, he admitted he was WRONG? Pasteur completely changed his mind and stated that the true cause of infection was NOT the germ, but the unhealthy condition of the body. In other words, Pasteur eventually recognised what Natural Health has taught for nearly 200 years, infection can only arise in those individuals whose body's are UNHEALTHY and TOXIC. It has been said that if the germ theory were true, there would be nobody left alive to believe it. That this theory still exists today, is for two reasons only, its commercial value to the drug and medical empires, and because the masses need something to blame for their self inflicted illnesses.

So where do germs fit in? As explained earlier, the germs true role in the body is to consume organic wastes undergoing putrefaction and decay. It stands to reason that the more toxic waste in your body, then the more germs you will have. In fact, germs are not our enemies, but our friends, for they are assisting in the important task of keeping the insides of our bodies clean. Germs, are like flies, they are attracted to filth, if you don't want germs, then get rid of the filth. Every time infection arises in the body, regardless of whether it's viral or bacterial, whether it's measles, herpes, veneral disease or even AIDS, the root cause of such infection, is in every case, an unhealthy toxic body. Whenever you read of so called epidemics of flu, or measles, or hepatitis, or AIDS, then realise this, those who succumb to these diseases do not possess healthy bodies.

By understanding the toxaemia theory and the true role of germs in the body, you will understand why Natural Health rejects the use of drugs and vaccines. Drugs do nothing to remove the toxic conditions of the body, the root cause of sickness. For this reason drugs cannot cure sickness, drugs merely suppress sickness. Treating bacterial infection with antibiotics kills the germs but doesn't remove the root cause of that infection, toxaemia. This is why it is so common for bacterial infection to continue to reoccur despite the lengthy use of antibiotics. Many mothers wonder why their children suffer recurrent ear or throat infections despite their children taking antibiotics. It is because drugs only suppress sickness, drugs do not cure sickness.

From his book, 'New Dimensions in Health', Dr. David Phillips writes:

"To believe that sickness results solely from the visitation of some itinerant germ or virus and to accept treatment by some poisonous drug is to be guilty of the most naive superstition. This form of exorcism cannot remedy the problem because it bears no relation to the real cause".

For the very same reason that drugs don't cure sickness, vaccines cannot prevent sickness. Vaccination is based on the idea that germs are the cause of sickness, and is aimed at giving protection against supposedly disease causing germs. Again, vaccination does not succeed in removing the toxic conditions of the body, and for this reason cannot prevent the development of infection within the body. This explains why vaccines are failing to prevent outbreaks of measles, whooping cough etc. In the industrialised countries, including Australia, anywhere between 50% to 95% of children who contract infectious disease have been previously fully vaccinated. In third world countries, millions have died from measles, diphtheria, polio, tuberculosis etc. despite being fully vaccinated. Like drugs, vaccines fail to remove the true underlying causes of disease, and for this reason, cannot and do not work.

By understanding the toxaemia theory and how sickness arises, you will understand the true means of disease prevention. If you don't want your children developing any of the infectious diseases, then you must ensure that their systems are kept clean and healthy. Remember, sickness only arises from a toxic system, if you wish to avoid sickness, then the system must be kept clean. If you don't want flies around the garbage bin, then keep the bin clean. If you don't want cockroaches in your cupboards, then keep your cupboards clean.

Now if sickness does arise in your child, if your child develops chicken pox, measles, whooping cough, etc., then realise that your child is experiencing a cleansing response, an elimination of toxic waste. Realise that this sickness serves a very important role in protecting the body from self-poisoning, and that it is therefore beneficial to the long term health of your child. Realise why under Natural Health treatment, no effort is made to drug the child's illness. Such illness is beneficial and is allowed to run it's course. The provision of bed rest, pure water, fresh air and quiet, is all the child needs, with the rewards being speedy recovery and better health in the child there afterwards.

"Illness or disease is only Nature's warning that filth has accumulated in some portion or other of the body, and it would be surely part of wisdom to allow Nature to remove the filth, instead of covering it up with the help of medicine. Those, therefore who take medicine only render the task of Nature more difficult".

Mahatma Gandhi

IMPORTANT NOTE

It is beyond the scope of this chapter (indeed this book) to give you a complete and thorough explanation of Natural Health theory. If Natural Health science is new to you, then no doubt you would have many questions about the toxaemia theory, the beneficial nature of acute illness and the non-drug treatment of disease. That is partly the purpose of this small book, to get you thinking, to challenge your beliefs, to expose erroneous medical theory and to stimulate your interest so that you be motivated to research further. Should you find the Natural Health philosophy on the prevention and treatment of disease appealing, then I encourage you to study further this philosophy so that you will have the confidence to put it into practise. If uncertainty exists, then seek out those health practitioners who embrace this philosophy in their clinical practices, or even better, seek out those persons who embrace this philosophy in their own lives, for they will be your best teachers.

"If a thousand old beliefs are ruined in our march to the truth, we must still march on".

5

VACCINATION
WHAT IT'S REALLY ABOUT

If vaccination doesn't work, if it doesn't protect our children from infectious disease, if it's dangerous and ineffective, then why are we told to vaccinate our children? Why are we told by our doctors, health authorities and government that if we don't vaccinate our children, then we are being irresponsible? Why are we told that our children can die, unless vaccinated? If vaccination does not work, then why are medical authorities pushing for compulsory vaccination?

To understand the true reasons behind the vaccination drive, you have to understand what the 'game' is all about. Vaccination is a multi-million dollar business under the complete control of the Drug Industry. Although the medical profession and government health departments administer all vaccination programs, they themselves are totally subservient to the drug industry because of financial arrangements. The medical profession receives millions in advertising revenue from the drug companies, and medical universities cannot operate without drug company funding. The drug industry also contribute millions of dollars to the political parties and even to political candidates thus ensuring favourable influence in government health policies and decisions.

Ever heard of the saying, *"he who pays the piper calls the tune"?* When it comes to vaccination, it is the drug industry who most definitely calls the tune. Their immense power, their infinite wealth, their control over medical education and the profession itself, their influence over government health policy and the mass media, it is these things that have enabled the drug industry to make vaccination a multi-million dollar bonanza. Eleanor McBean PhD (The Poisoned Needle) writes: *"The vaccine business has continued to thrive in spite of its disastrous failure, for the mere reason that it nets millions of dollars for the promoters, and this buys power with governments and propaganda control over the masses who don't know how to think for themselves".*

This does not mean however that the medical profession or government health departments can plead innocence to their own involvement in the promotion of vaccination. The medical profession has achieved much of its power and prestige by convincing the masses that vaccination is what saved us all. If the medical profession are to hold on to their power, they cannot allow the masses to discover the truth, to discover that improved hygiene, nutrition and sanitation are what really saved us, and not vaccination as claimed. They cannot allow the masses to find out about the many hundreds of studies linking vaccination to childhood illness, asthma, skin disease, juvenile diabetes, behavioural disorders, leukaemia and cancers, all of which have risen dramatically since the era of vaçcination commenced. The medical profession, if they wish to retain their power and prestige, have no choice but to continue deluding the people into believing in the necessity and importance of vaccination.

As far as the government goes, they haven't much choice either. Think about it, they have been telling everyone for fifty years that vaccines are safe and effective. They can hardly turn around now and admit they were wrong. The government have dug themselves a hole from which they cannot get out. What politician is going to stand on the public platform and admit that vaccines do not really work after all? What politician is going to publicly admit that Cot Deaths can be caused by the triple antigen vaccine, one of the vaccines that the government offers free to all children? Vaccination has become a runaway train which they cannot stop.

Now I am not accusing all doctors, nurses, health workers and those involved in the administering of vaccines as being a party to the sinister motives behind vaccination. Most orthodox health professionals are totally ignorant of the overwhelming evidence exposing the dangers and ineffectiveness of vaccines. They are however, very much like well trained soldiers, they follow orders without question. This, along with the medical indoctrination they are subject to in their training, ensures their loyal service. Few will escape this process, and of those who do, most will be afraid to speak out. Such is the system.

Let us have a brief look at how the Authorities (Drug, Medical and Government) coerce the population into believing in and accepting vaccinations.

Firstly, they tell us that there are all these germs (bacteria and viruses) that can kill our children. If they do not kill them, they can cause horrible complications and long term suffering.

Secondly, they have us believe that we have absolutely no power to protect ourselves from these deadly germs or killer diseases. They tell us that no matter how healthy we are, we can still die from these diseases, and that therefore, health is no protection.

Thirdly, they tell us that our only chance of survival, our only possibility of protection, is from their drugs and vaccines, that we have to BUY. (your taxes are paying for them).

Now I am pretty sure that you dear reader can see the game. I doubt if you would be reading this book otherwise. Unfortunately, most people do not see the game. This is because most people do not think for themselves, nor do they question what they are told. Instead, they listen to the authorities and accept what they are told as 'truth'. The amazing thing about it, is that whilst they easily accept such fraudulent information, they will not so easily dispose of it. In fact, many will go to their graves defending it, despite all proof to the contrary. A good example of human nature at it's worst.

Another reason why the majority are so quick to accept vaccinations is that it removes their responsibility. If you vaccinate your child, then should your child get sick, you will not be held responsible. No one can blame you because you did the right thing. Most people avoid responsibility like they avoid the plague.

One of the most powerful means of manipulating people and controlling them is through FEAR. Tell the people that they are at the mercy of killer germs, and that their only protection is drugs and vaccines, and you've got them. Millions of them will line up for their shots, like sheep to the slaughter.

So through propaganda, lies and scare tactics, about 90% of the population are sucked in to vaccinating. What of the other 10%? Well about half of these will eventually succumb to the pressure that vaccine promoters exert upon them to vaccinate. For example, *could you live with yourself if your child died of a disease which you could have prevented through vaccination?* Or, *you are putting the community and other children at risk from your un-vaccinated child.* Or, *if you do not vaccinate, then you are committing child abuse,* etc. etc. This sort of pressure, is difficult to withstand if you do not have the knowledge and understanding of the whole subject.

So by this stage you have got 95% of the population vaccinated. Now in case you didn't know, the vaccination rate in Australia is pretty close to 95% at the present time. The medical authorities will not admit to this and claim a vaccination rate of only 50%, but I can assure all readers that this is not true. Over the past year I have travelled throughout the Eastern States of Australia and have given vaccination seminars in over 95 towns. Having spoken to many hundreds of parents, practitioners and health workers, it is still, at this point in time, only a minority who are not vaccinating their children. I visited many towns and cities where parents admitted that their own children were the only ones in their school un-vaccinated. In most cases parents admit to having very little support from their communities or schools, and are continually being pressured and harassed over their refusal to vaccinate their children. Many parents simply keep silent. Having said all this, yes I agree awareness about the ineffectiveness and dangers of vaccination is growing, but just realise that it is still only a minority that have this awareness.

Now medical authorities in alliance with the drug industry, are not satisfied with a 95% vaccination rate, they want 100%. If the truth be known, they would like every man, women and child in this country to be fully vaccinated, and to achieve this, they are endeavouring to introduce the most effective tactic by far - COMPULSORY VACCINATION. This has happened in America and many a parent who have refused vaccination for their children have been charged with child abuse. So why the push for compulsory vaccination?

Authorities will claim that with everyone vaccinated, outbreaks of infectious disease will not occur and so our children will be safe. This has proven false with major outbreaks of measles and whooping cough regularly occurring amongst fully vaccinated children in the United States. These outbreaks have been well documented in the Journal of the American Medical Association. One article on measles (JAMA 21/11/90) states *"Although more than 95% of school-aged children in the United States are vaccinated against measles, large measles outbreaks continue to occur in schools, and most cases in this setting occur among previously vaccinated children"*.

In fact there is a history of disease outbreaks in population groups subject to compulsory vaccination going back 150 years. The biggest smallpox disasters with the highest mortality rates occurred in England, Germany, Philippines, Japan, Italy and several other countries AFTER smallpox vaccination was made compulsory.

The way I see it, there are several reasons for pushing compulsory vaccination;

1. Increased profit to the Drug Companies.

2. By making vaccination compulsory, it will reinforce in people's minds that vaccines must work. *"Why would they make vaccination compulsory if it did not work?"* the people will ask.

3. By vaccinating every child, it will be even more difficult to prove vaccine-induced illness in children, because there will be no un-vaccinated children to compare them with. For example, according to a London study (reported in the Herald Sun, September 14 and 20, 1994) asthma occurred five times more frequently in vaccinated children than those not vaccinated. This observation was only possible by comparing a vaccinated group with an un-vaccinated group. If all children are vaccinated, no such comparison can be made, and therefore no observable link to vaccine-induced illness.

4. IGNORANCE. The great majority of doctors and health officials, ignorant of the evidence exposing the dangers and ineffectiveness of vaccines, actually ***believe*** that vaccines are safe and effective and therefore see compulsory vaccination as a necessary safeguard.

There is one other possible motive behind the push for compulsory vaccination. When you vaccinate a population group, you make them weaker, this is a provable physiological fact. Now according to conspiracy theorists, weakening population groups renders them less resistant to totalitarian rule. Too over the top you reckon, personally, I am not so sure. In World War 2, a number of German and Russian POW camps were putting a substance into the prisoners drinking water to keep them docile and more accepting of authority. What was the substance? FLUORIDE.

One thing for sure, vaccination is a crime of the greatest magnitude. In the two hundred year history of vaccinations, the lay public have been deceived, mislead and downright lied to. Unfortunately, as Adolf Hitler once said,

"When you tell a lie loud enough, often enough and big enough, the people will eventually believe it".

6

QUESTIONS AND ANSWERS

Here are some of the most common questions I am asked at vaccination seminars and my answers to them. I emphasise that my answers do not constitute 'advice' but merely my current beliefs and opinions. It is up to each reader to formulate their own beliefs and determine their own course of action.

Question What's your opinion of Homeopathic Prophylaxis? (often referred to as Homeopathic Vaccination)

Answer This is a controversial question for even amongst Homeopaths, there is widespread disagreement as to its validity and efficacy. My answer to this question is based upon my understanding of the causes and nature of disease, and human physiology. I firmly believe that illness in children, particularly the infectious diseases, can only arise if their bodies are toxic and polluted. It stands to reason therefore, that if you wish to prevent illness in children you must keep their bodies clean and hygienic, or in other words, in physiological health. This is only possible by embracing the laws of health as explained in Chapter 2. In those children that do possess a clean system, who do possess physiological health, I would ask, why would they need homeopathic prophylaxis.? If they are truly healthy, then they cannot and will not get sick. They don't need protection, they already have it - HEALTH.

Now in those children who are not healthy, whose systems are polluted, whose bloodstream's are toxic, I would again ask, why would they need homeopathic prophylaxis? Why would you want to prevent these children from developing measles, whooping cough, chicken pox etc. Remember, these diseases serve to eliminate toxic waste from the system, they are BENEFICIAL, they cleanse the body, thereby restoring health. These sicknesses are not evil, they are not germs attacking the body, they are in fact, well regulated physiological actions, having as their objective, the protection of the bodies cells and tissues. Children who develop acute illness, including the infectious diseases, and treated in accordance with Natural Health principles, will be in better health afterwards.

I well realise that many parents will have a hard time accepting this philosophy. For most of us, we have been so conditioned to drugs and vaccines, that the idea of not needing them, or not using them, is initially hard to accept. Many parents turn to Homeopathy because they feel they still must do something, they must give their children a remedy to help or protect them. Their actions are motivated more by fear, ignorance and hope, than by understanding and comprehension. I'm certainly not telling parents to avoid Homeopaths, on the contrary, go to your Homeopaths, examine their philosophy, question their ideas on disease causation, question their views on treating disease, and examine and verify the evidence supporting Homeopathy.

Then, by understanding the basic philosophies of Natural Health, Homeopathy and Orthodox Medicine, you will be in the best position to make your own informed decisions.

Question You say fever in children is beneficial, can't fever cause brain damage and death?

Answer Firstly, you must realise that the symptoms of infectious disease, fever, inflammation, vomiting, skin rashes, etc. do not constitute the disease but the effects. The real disease is Toxaemia, the symptoms represent the efforts of the body to eliminate toxic waste, and are therefore beneficial. With fever, there is an inbuilt mechanism within the brain to ensure that it does not reach dangerous levels (only where suppressive treatment is employed, or when the patient refuses to rest, does fever have the potential to become dangerous). This is why under Natural Health, no attempt is made to treat or suppress these symptoms. Instead, by allowing them to run their course, the body is cleansed of toxic waste.

It stands to reason that if you attempt to suppress or stop these symptoms, fever in particular, then you are basically preventing the body from cleansing itself. The body is forced to retain the poisonous waste matter that it is struggling to remove. When this happens, you are indeed creating the potential for damage and complications to occur. If you were to examine the case history of any child who died or suffered complications from having a fever, you will find that the child, in most cases, was treated with suppressive drug therapy. What I am saying, is that in most, if not all cases where children have suffered complications or damages from infectious disease, the causes are due to suppressive drugs and wrong treatment. In many cases, you will also find a history of poor health or underlying illness in the child.

I will not say that it has never happened, but in ten years of research, I have never come across a case of a child who has suffered any complications or damage from an infectious disease when treated in accordance with Natural Health principles. I firmly believe that drug therapy and suppressive treatment is the true cause for complications and life threatening episodes.

Question What about children who have been vaccine damaged, don't they need some sort of medicine or remedy to fix them?

Answer Realise this, the human body is a self-maintaining, self-regulating and self-healing mechanism. If the body has been damaged or poisoned in any way the body will do everything in its power to fix itself. If the problem is fixable, if the vaccine damage is repairable, if the broken part is healable, then as long as there is sufficient VITALITY, the body will heal, the body will fix the problem, it will repair the damage. Most people think that when something is wrong with the body, then some sort of medicine or remedy is needed to fix it. All that is needed is sufficient vitality or life-force, for this is the only power that the body requires in order to carry out its repairs. If the damage is not fixable, if it is beyond repair, then nothing can fix it, no matter how many remedies are given.

From the Natural Health viewpoint, if a child is vaccine damaged, then do everything to support and enhance its vitality, ensure correct spinal alignment and muscular balance, detoxify the child's body through cleansing diets, expose the child's naked body to fresh air and sunshine, give the child pure water, rest and comfort, and above all else, be as loving and caring towards the child as you can. These are the means to raise and enhance the vitality of the child, thus providing the best chance of recovery from illness and vaccine damage.

The body has tremendous powers of regeneration and restoration, but it is wholly dependent upon adequate nerve force and healing power (vitality) and whether or not the damage is repairable.

Question Are you saying that you should never take medical drugs for your sickness?

Answer One of the biggest critics of modern medicine was a doctor from its own ranks, Dr. Robert Mendelsohn. He stated that if you took all the medicine on earth and threw it in the ocean, it would be all the better for mankind and all the worst for the fishes. Drugs do not cure sickness, drugs do not make you healthier, drugs possess no power of their own, drugs are poisonous to the biological system, drugs weaken vitality. Their only justifiable use in my mind, is in certain life-threatening conditions such as anaphylactic shock, severe asthmatic attacks, respiratory failure, heart attack, septic shock etc. So I do not condemn the use of medical drugs outright, I am not suggesting that medical attention should not be sought when ill. Medical diagnosis has a valuable role to play, and emergency medical treatment for acute emergencies and accident victims is second to none.

But I am saying this, if you or your children suffer from any of the acute or chronic illnesses such as colds, flu, infectious disease, asthma, skin disease, hay fever, arthritis etc., the use of medical drugs, although giving short term relief, will ultimately worsen your health. This is because drugs fail to remove the underlying causes of illness (toxaemia) and because of the toxic effects of the drugs themselves. If you really value your own and your children's health, then I would urge you to thoroughly study and understand Natural Health philosophy. By doing so you will know when to take drugs and when not to, you will know when to visit a doctor and when not to, and above all, you will know how to maintain the health of your children, so that they never need drugs in the first place.

Question Medical Authorities claim that the benefits of vaccination far outway its risks. What do you think?

Answer What benefits? How can vaccination convey any benefits when it doesn't work? The injection of foreign poisonous material (vaccines) into the human bloodstream does nothing to strengthen the body, but everything to weaken it. Make no mistake, vaccination has never been of benefit to so much as one single human being, on the contrary in the two hundred year history of vaccinations, millions have died because of its poisonous and destructive effects. The risks of vaccination can never be justified because vaccines should never be employed in the first place.

Question Must my children be vaccinated in order to be enrolled at school?

Answer At the time of this writing (January 1995) I am not aware of any laws which state children must be vaccinated prior to school entry. However I am aware that authorities are endeavouring to create that impression by warning that children will be refused entry into schools unless vaccinated. In fact, all that schools require is a certificate which you fill out indicating whether the child has been vaccinated or not. Should an outbreak of infectious disease occur, unvaccinated children will be required to stay home until the school outbreak is over. According to the authorities, this ensures the safety of the vaccinated children.

Question What can be done to stop vaccination becoming compulsory?

Answer Firstly, I doubt whether the government will actually legislate for compulsory vaccination. If they do they will have to introduce a compensation act to cover children damaged by vaccines. This has happened in America and has cost the government millions. I may be wrong, but that is how I see it at present. The Australian Government are not keen on forking out payments to vaccine damaged children, so they may hold off on making vaccination compulsory. They will however continue the propaganda in favour of vaccination, and encourage all children to be vaccinated.

On the other hand should the government attempt to legislate compulsory vaccination, then every effort must be made to inform the lay public of the dangers and ineffectiveness of vaccines. This is already happening with the formation of vaccine information groups around the country. These groups are now providing parents and the public with information on the true risks associated with vaccines and their ineffectiveness. The more people who find out the truth, then the less chance the government will have of forcing vaccination upon us.

This is where you can help. I have included a vaccination information sheet at the back of this book which you can photocopy and hand out to friends and family. Also, whenever you are confronted by doctors, nurses, health workers, well meaning friends etc., all telling you how important vaccination is, then simply give them a copy of this sheet. You should realise that most doctors, nurses, etc. are not aware of these facts, so by offering them the vaccine information sheet, you will be sowing the seeds of awareness. Do not back down from those telling you to vaccinate, you have the facts and the truth, you must stand up to those who would push vaccinations. Remember, you are fighting to preserve the health of our children, you have the truth, therefore you have the POWER.

"Evil occurs, because good people sit back and do nothing"

VACCINATION INFORMATION SHEET

DID YOU KNOW .....

--- That up to 90% of the decline in death rates from infectious disease occurred BEFORE vaccination commenced.

--- That in the UK, since 1970, more than 200,000 cases of whooping cough have occurred in fully vaccinated children.

--- That in the US, despite compulsory vaccination, measles is on the increase and many outbreaks are occurring amongst fully vaccinated children.

--- That a tuberculosis vaccine trial in India involving over 260,000 Indians resulted in more TB cases in the vaccinated than the un-vaccinated.

--- That almost every polio case in the US in the last 30 years has been associated with the vaccine itself, the same vaccine given to all Australian children.

--- The cost of the whooping cough vaccine had risen from 11 cents in 1982 to $11.40 in 1987. The Vaccine company was putting aside $8.00 per shot to cover legal costs and damages being paid out to parents of brain damaged children and children who die after vaccination.

--- About the contaminated polio vaccines given to millions of children in the early 1960's. These vaccines contained the SV 40 virus which causes cancer in animals, as well as changes in human cell tissue cultures.

--- That America's No 1 AIDS researcher, Dr. Robert Gallo has speculated that the AIDS explosion was triggered by the World Health Organisation's smallpox campaign throughout Africa, Haiti and Brazil.

--- That a survey in the UK involving 600 Doctors revealed that 50% of them refused the Hepatitis B Vaccine despite belonging to the high risk group urged to be vaccinated. Amongst the reasons given for their refusal were *"I do not trust the vaccine"* and *"Vaccination is of no proven benefit"*.

--- That in 1976 Dr. Anthony Morris, former chief vaccine control officer of the US Food and Drug Administration was "sacked" for warning the American public about the dangers of the flu vaccine.

--- That Britain's leading vaccine manufacturer, the Wellcome Company were forced to cease vaccine production. The reasons cited by their company spokesman Dr. A.J Beale were "too much litigation's and too little profit".

--- That in the U.S., from July 1990 to November 1993, the US Food and Drug Administration counted a total of 54,072 adverse reactions following vaccination. The FDA admitted that this number represented only 10% of the real total, because most doctors were refusing to report vaccine injuries. In other words, adverse reactions for this period exceeded half a million.

www.vaccinationdebate.com

DOCTORS CONDEMN VACCINATION

"The greatest threat of childhood disease lies in the dangerous and ineffectual efforts made to prevent them through mass immunisation".

Dr. R. Mendelsohn
Author and Paediatrician

"Official data have shown that the large-scale vaccinations undertaken in the US have failed to obtain any significant improvement of the diseases against which they were supposed to provide protection".

Dr. A. Sabin
Developer of Polio Vaccine

"There is a great deal of evidence to prove that immunisation of children does more harm than good".

Dr. Anthony Morris
Research Scientist

"In our opinion, there is now sufficient evidence of immune malfunction following current vaccination programs to anticipate growing public demands for research investigation into alternative methods of prevention of infectious disease".

Dr's. H. Buttram and J. Hoffman
Vaccinations and Immune Malfunctions

"In addition to the many obvious cases of mortality from these practices, there are also long-term hazards which are almost impossible to estimate accurately ..... the inherent danger of all vaccine procedures should be a deterrent to their unnecessary or unjustifiable use".

Sir Graham Wilson
The Hazards of Immunisation

"Every vaccine carries certain hazards and can produce inward reactions in some people ..... in general, there are more vaccine complications than is generally appreciated".

Professor George Dick
London University

"Laying aside the very real possibility that the various vaccines are contaminated with animal viruses and may cause serious illness later in life (multiple sclerosis, cancer, leukaemia, kreutzfeld-jacob disease, etc.) we must consider whether the vaccines really work for the intended purpose".

Dr. William Campbell Douglas
Cutting Edge, May 1990

"All vaccination has the effect of directing the three values of the blood into or toward the zone characteristics of cancer and leukaemia ..... Vaccines DO predispose to cancer and leukaemia".

Professor L.C. Vincent
Founder of Bioelectronics

"Many here voice a silent view that the Salk and Sabin polio vaccine, being made of monkey kidney tissue has been directly responsible for the major increase in leukaemia in this country".

Dr. Frederick Klenner
Polio Researcher, USA